Nutrifitness

Volume II

Traditional Medicines and Herbal Medications

Acknowledgements

I wish to thank my friend Zena Enlow who pushed me to write this follow-up to Nutrifitness.
Sarah and Heather Morey my beautiful granddaughters, I hope this will help your future. Thanks to my wife Gery Morey for her great editorial assistance.

Introduction

For many generations traditional medicines and herbs have been used for treating many illnesses and afflictions. Many people in the East, and the indigenous people of North America used, and still use many of these medications.

A large percentage of our pharmacopoeia is made up of herbal products. It is time we learn about these medicines, and combine them with our fine western medicines. These medicinals were researched when writing *Nutrifitness.*

Let us explore these products.

Flaxseed Oil (Linseed Oil)

Flaxseed oil is derived from the Flax plant. Flaxseed Oil and Flaxseed contain substances that promote good health. One of these substances is alpha-linolenic acid (ALA), an essential fatty acid that appears to be beneficial for heart disease, inflammatory bowel disease, arthritic, and other health conditions. Flaxseed, in addition to ALA, contains a group of chemicals called Lignans that may play a role in the prevention of Cancer.

ALA, as well as eicosapentanoic acid (EPA) and Docahexanoic acid (DHA) belong to substances called omega-3 fatty acids, Although similar in structure, the benefits of ALA, EPA, and DHA are not necessarily the same. Fish should also be an important part of the diet, or supplements of EPA and DHA should be taken.

Clinical studies indicate that Flaxseed oil and other omega-3 fatty acids may be helpful in treating a variety of diseases. The evidence is strongest for heart disease.

Flaxseed oil is available in liquid and soft-gel capsule forms. Flaxseed oil may turn rancid if it is not refrigerated. Flaxseed oil requires special packaging because it is easily destroyed by heat, light and oxygen. The highest quality are manufactured using fresh pressed seeds, bottled in dark or opaque containers, and processed at low temperatures in the absence of light, heat and oxygen.

Kava-Kava Root

If you have had the chance to visit Hawaii or one of the other islands in the South Pacific, there's a good chance you've come in contact with Kava Kava. Kava is an essential and integral part of life in the Pacific Islands often thought of as one of the most precious gifts from the Earth. Not only is it a pleasant drink that can be a safe alternative to alcohol, but also Kava Kava has been prescribed as an effective folk remedy for anxiety, insomnia and back pain.

My response to its use has been highly positive, in my bouts with insomnia. It relaxes me, and makes me quite calm. I mix it as a tea in the evening.

Kava Root (the only part of the plant that is used) is largely employed as a celebratory drink much in the same way that alcohol is used in the West. It helps mark momentous occasions such as weddings, public festivals, political powwows and holidays, and it is even used in ceremonies honoring the dead. Unlike alcohol, kava does not produce or stimulate aggression. It does not condemn the user to a dreaded hangover, unlike alcohol. Alcohol literally kills hundreds of thousands of people a year, and Kava, when properly harvested, has never actually hurt anyone. Kava has even been known to help reduce alcohol consumption!

Many people find other uses for kava, including many medicinal ones. It's interesting to note that kava has been shown to help ease anxiety, depression as well as producing a restful sleep. Athletes, businessmen and diplomats to help "take the edge off" and focus concentration use it. Widely prescribed throughout Oceania and Europe to treat hyperactivity in children, it has also been used to aid children who have difficulty sleeping on occasion.

Kava has not been shown to be addictive, and has been safely used for over 3000 years.
Kava can:
1. Relax Muscles
2. Calm Nerves
3. Create a feeling of well-being
4. Induce a feeling of peace
5. Has been used as an Herbal aphrodisiac
6. reduces inhibitions, and makes people more sociable

In the South Pacific, drinking kava is mostly used for ceremonial, recreational and social purposes. Kava is consumed at the end of the workday, and the ritual of kava preparation and drinking provides one with both an opportunity for individual meditation as well as a social time. With inhibitions alleviated.

In our hectic, modern society "kava time" is anytime. The fact that kava does not slow one's mental capacity that allows it to be used during the day especially when we find ourselves anxious or in stressful situations like:
1. Going on a date
2. Visiting the Dentist
3. Giving a presentation
4. Attending a party
5. Enhance athletic abilities
6. Taking an exam

And for the most part, kava is best consumed after work when the kava's delightful, pleasurable, relaxing effects can be experienced while one is able to relax into a happy, peaceful state with complete mental alertness. When kava is taken before bedtime, it induces a restful sleep and encourages a refreshed feeling upon awakening.

Kava has no side effects when taken in moderate doses, although its abuse can lead to health problems. A study of heavy abusers in the South Pacific showed evidence of shortness of breath, dry scaly skin, and slight alterations in red and white blood cells and platelets. The reports of liver damage have widely been dismissed – it was one irresponsible kava manufacturer, which used the poisonous tops of the kava plant in one of their products that lead to the liver damage. Even the country that hosted the study (Germany) has repealed their ban on Kava Kava because it has been proven a safe and effective herbal product.

The most significant anti-anxiety studies show that an effective daily dose of kava is 70-210 milligrams of kavalactones. The amount of kava to take depends on your purpose for using it and your individual sensitivity to the effects of kavalactones.

Death or severe illness from exclusive use of kava has not been reported in any medical literature.

Whenever you first try a new medicine, herb or supplement, it is always best to start with low dosages and builds up. Kava, if used appropriately, can reduce the stress in our daily lives, as well as alleviate the amount of anxiety one might anticipate becoming exposed to, such as in a stressful negotiation. Studies show the occasional use of kava presents no health problems. Years of use in Germany have produced no reports of troublesome drug interactions as well.

If you have any questions or concerns about your health or possible interactions with prescription medications, simply consult your doctor.

Many people find other medicinal uses for kava kava. It is interesting to note that kava has been shown to help ease anxiety and depression, as well as help induce a restful sleep. Athletes as well as businessmen to help "take the edge off" and focus concentration use it.

Dong-Quai

Dong quai

Dong quai (Angelica sinensis) root has been used for more than a thousand years as a spice, tonic, and medicine in China, Korea, and Japan. It is still used often in traditional Chinese medicine (TCM), where it is usually combined with other herbs. In TCM it is used most often to treat women's reproductive problems, such as dysmenorrhea (painful menstruation), and to improve circulation. Dong quai is sometimes called the "female ginseng." Although there are few scientific studies on dong quai, it is sometimes suggested to relieve menstrual disorders such as cramps, irregular menstrual cycles, infrequent periods, premenstrual syndrome (PMS), and menopausal symptoms.

Dong quai grows at high altitudes in the cold, damp, mountains of China, Korea, and Japan. This fragrant, perennial plant -- a member of the celery family -- has smooth purplish stems and bears umbrella-shaped clusters of white flowers and winged fruits in July and August. The yellowish-brown thick-branched roots of the dong quai plant have several medicinal uses. It takes 3 years for the plant to reach maturity, after which the root is harvested and formulated into tablets, powders, and other medicinal forms.

Dong quai is sometimes suggested for the following conditions:

Menopausal symptoms

Some women report relief of symptoms such as hot flashes when taking dong quai. Researchers aren't sure whether dong quai has estrogen-like effects or if it blocks estrogens in the body, and the studies so far have been conflicting. One study found that dong quai did not help to relieve menopausal symptoms.

Dong quai has also been suggested for these conditions, although scientific evidence is lacking:

Amenorrhea (absence of menstruation)

Heart disease -- One study suggested that when used in combination with Asian ginseng (Panax ginseng) and astragalus (Astragalus membranaceus), dong quai decreased symptoms of chest pain in a small group of people with heart disease.

High blood pressure

Precautions:

You should not drink the essential oil of dong quai because it contains a small amount of cancer-causing substances.

Those who have chronic diarrhea or abdominal bloating should not use dong quai. People who are at risk of hormone-related cancers, including breast, ovarian, and uterine cancers, should not take dong quai because researchers aren't sure if it has estrogen-like effects.

Dong quai, particularly at high doses, may increase your sensitivity to sunlight and cause skin inflammation and rashes. Stay out of the sun or use sunscreen while taking dong quai.

Dong quai should not be used during pregnancy because it may cause the uterus to contract and raise the risk of miscarriage. Nursing mothers should avoid dong quai because information on its safety is lacking.

Children should not take dong quai because information on its safety is lacking.

Dong quai may interact with the following medications and herbs:

Anticoagulants (blood-thinners) -- Dong quai may increase the effects of these drugs, including warfarin (Coumadin), and raise the risk of bleeding. The same is true of using dong quai with the herbs listed below. Talk to your doctor before taking dong quai with any of the following:

Feverfew (Tanacetum parthenium)

Garlic (Allium sativum)

Ginger (Zingiber officinale)

Ginkgo (Ginkgo biloba)

Ginseng (Panax ginseng)

Licorice (Glycyrrhiza glabra)

Chinese skullcap (Scutellaria baicalensis)

Turmeric (Curcuma longa)

Hormone medications -- There is little research on using dong quai with hormone medications -- such as estrogens, progesterones, oral contraceptives, tamoxifen, or raloxifene. But, because dong quai may have estrogen-like effects, you should not take it with hormone medications except under your doctor's supervision.

St. John's wort -- Both dong quai and St. John's wort can increase your sensitivity to sunlight. Talk to your doctor before use.

Milk Thistle

Health benefits

For many centuries extracts of milk thistle have been recognized as "liver tonics.". Research into the biological activity of silymarin and its possible medical uses has been conducted in many countries since the 1970s, but the quality of the research has been uneven. Milk thistle has been reported to have protective effects on the liver and to greatly improve its function. It is typically used to treat liver cirrhosis, chronic hepatitis (liver inflammation), toxin-induced liver damage (including the prevention of severe liver damage from Amanita phalloides (death cap) mushroom poisoning), and gallbladder disorders. Reviews of the literature covering clinical studies of silymarin vary in their conclusions. A review using only studies with both double-blind and placebo protocols concluded that milk thistle and its derivatives "does not seem to significantly influence the course of patients with alcoholic and/or hepatitis B or C liver diseases." A different review of the literature, performed for the U. S. Department of Health and Human Services, found that, while there is strong evidence of legitimate medical benefits, the studies done to date are of such uneven design and quality that no firm conclusions about degrees of effectiveness for specific conditions or appropriate dosage can yet be made. A review of studies of silymarin and liver disease which are available on the web shows an interesting pattern in that studies which tested low dosages of silymarin concluded that silymarin was ineffective, while studies which used significantly larger doses concluded that silymarin was biologically active and had therapeutic effects.

Toxin-induced liver damage

Research suggests that milk thistle extracts both prevent and repair damage to the liver from toxic chemicals and medications. Workers who had been exposed to vapors from toxic chemicals (toluene and/or xylene) for 5-20 years were given either a standardized milk thistle extract (80% silymarin) or placebo for 30 days. The workers taking the milk thistle extract showed significant improvement in liver function tests (ALT and AST) and platelet counts vs. the placebo group.

The efficacy of silymarin in preventing drug-induced liver damage in patients taking psychotropic drugs long-term has been investigated .

This class of drugs is known to cause liver damage from oxidation of lipids. Patients taking silymarin in the study had less hepatic damage from the oxidation of lipids than patients taking the placebo.

In a 2009 study published in the journal Cancer, milk thistle showed promise in reducing the liver damaging effects of chemotherapy in a study of 50 children.

Amanita mushroom poisoning

The efficacy of thirty different treatments was analyzed in a retrospective study of 205 cases of Amanita phalloides (death cap) mushroom poisoning.[Both penicillin and hyperbaric oxygen independently contributed to a higher rate of survival. When silybin [silibinin] was added to the penicillin treatment, survival was increased even more. In another 18 cases of death cap poisoning, a correlation was found between the time elapsed before initiation of silybin therapy, and the severity of the poisoning. The data indicates that severe liver damage in Amanita phalloides poisoning can be prevented effectively when administration of silybin begins within 48 hours of mushroom intake. In a recent 2007 event, a family of six was treated with milk thistle and a combination of other treatments to save them from ingested poisonous mushrooms. While five of the six made a full recovery, the grandmother showed liver recovery but was overcome by kidney failure related to the poisonous mushrooms. Other uses

Beside benefits for liver disease, other treatment claims include:

Used as a post (oral steroid) cycle therapy for body builders] and/or in the hopes of reducing or eliminating liver damage

Lowering cholesterol levels

Reducing insulin resistance in people with type 2 diabetes who also have cirrhosis

Reducing the growth of cancer cells in breast, cervical, and prostate cancers

Used in many products claiming to reduce the effects of a hangover.

Used by individuals withdrawing from opiates, especially during the Acute Withdrawal Stage.

Used by those taking oral steroids

Reducing liver damaging from Chemotherapeutic agents

Cayenne Pepper

Cayenne PepperCapsicum frutescensFam: SolanaceaeCayenne pepper takes its name from its supposed centre of origin - the Cayenne region of French Guiana, Cayenne deriving from a Tupi Indian name. It is now grown largely in India, East Africa, Mexico and the United States, in fact most tropical and sub-tropical regions. Chiles originated in South America, where they have been under cultivation since prehistoric times. The seed's long viability facilitated the rapid spread of the plant throughout the tropics and sub-tropics by the Spanish and Portuguese, the spice becoming as popular there as vine pepper. Chiles were long known as 'Indian' pepper - meaning 'of the New World' rather than 'of India'. Despite its specific name, and the supposed use of special chiles for it, there is little to distinguish cayenne from ordinary pure chilli powder, except that commercial 'chilli powder' usually contains other spices such as garlic or cumin, and is rougher in texture.

Attributed Medicinal Properties

Cayenne pepper exerts a number of beneficial effects on the cardiovascular system. It reduces the likelihood of developing arteriosclerosis by reducing blood cholesterol and triglyceride levels. Cayenne also reduces the platelet aggregation and increases fibrinolytic activity. Cultures consuming a large amount of Cayenne pepper have a much lower rate of cardiovascular disease. Cayenne has been used as medicine for centuries. It was considered helpful for various conditions of the gastrointestinal tract, including stomachaches, cramping pains, and gas. Cayenne was frequently used to treat diseases of the circulatory system. It is still traditionally used in herbal medicine as a circulatory tonic (a substance believed to improve circulation). Rubbed onto the skin, Cayenne is a traditional, as well as modern, remedy for rheumatic pains and arthritis due to what is termed as a "counterirritant" effect. A counterirritant is something that causes irritation to a tissue to which it is applied, thus distracting from the original irritation (such as joint pain in the case of arthritis). Many people consume lots of hot peppers in tropical climates as the heat will induce perspiration, which actually helps a person to cool off. Cayenne's primary chemical constituents include capsaicin, capsanthine, beta carotene, flavonoids, and vitamin C. Cayenne causes the brain to secrete more endorphins. It is considered thermogenic, meaning it can "rev up" metabolism and aid in weight loss. Cayenne also improves circulation. Cayenne helps to relieve pain, not only due to its endorphin enhancing properties.

Chamomile

Chamomile has been used medicinally for thousands of years and is widely used in Europe. It is a popular treatment for numerous ailments, including sleep disorders, anxiety, digestion/intestinal conditions, skin infections/inflammation (including eczema), wound healing, infantile colic, teething pains, and diaper rash. In the United States, chamomile is best known as an ingredient in herbal tea preparations advertised for mild sedating effects. German chamomile (Matricaria recutita) and Roman chamomile (Chamaemelum nobile) are the two major types of chamomile used for health conditions. They are believed to have similar effects on the body, although German chamomile may be slightly stronger. Most research has used German chamomile, which is more commonly used everywhere except for England, where Roman chamomile is more common.

Although chamomile is widely used, there is not enough reliable research in humans to support its use for any condition. Despite its reputation as a gentle medicinal plant, there are many reports of allergic reactions in people after eating or coming into contact with chamomile preparations, including life-threatening anaphylaxis.

Chamomile may increase the amount of drowsiness caused by some herbs or supplements. Caution is advised while driving or operating machinery.

In theory, chamomile may increase the risk of bleeding when taken with other products that are believed to increase the risk of bleeding. Multiple cases of bleeding have been reported with the use of Ginkgo biloba , and fewer cases with garlic and saw palmetto. Numerous other agents may theoretically increase the risk of bleeding, although this has not been proven in most cases.

Chamomile may interfere with the way the body processes certain drugs using the liver's "cytochrome P450" enzyme system. As a result, the levels of other herbs or supplements may become too high in the blood. It may also alter the effects that other herbs or supplements possibly have on the P450 system. Patients using any medications should check the package insert and speak with a healthcare professional including a pharmacist about possible interactions.

Chamomile may have anti-estrogenic effects and interact with herbs and supplements like red clover or soy.

Based on preliminary study, constituents in chamomile may alter blood sugar or blood pressure. Patients taking herbs or supplements that affect blood sugar or blood pressure should be cautious.

Chamomile may have anti-inflammatory effects. Theoretically, the use of chamomile with other anti-inflammatory herbs and supplements may have additive effects.

Chamomile may interact with herbs and supplements that act as cardiac depressants, cardiac glycosides, respiratory depressants, or spasmolytics.

Chamomile may also interact with antibacterial, antifungal, antihistamine, or diuretic herbs and supplements, as well as herbs and supplements used for high cholesterol, ulcers, diarrhea, or gastrointestinal disorders.

Turmeric or Curcumin

Turmeric has been used historically as a component of Indian Ayurvedic medicine since 1900 BCE to treat a wide variety of ailments. Research in the latter half of the 20th century has identified curcumin as responsible for most of the biological activity of turmeric. In vitro and animal studies have suggested a wide range of potential therapeutic or preventive effects associated with curcumin. At present, these effects have not been confirmed in humans. However, as of 2008, numerous clinical trials in humans were underway, studying the effect of curcumin on numerous diseases including multiple myeloma, pancreatic cancer, myelodysplastic syndromes, colon cancer, psoriasis, and Alzheimer's disease.

In vitro and animal studies have suggested that curcumin may have antitumor, antioxidant, antiarthritic, anti-amyloid, anti-ischemic, and anti-inflammatory properties. Anti-inflammatory properties may be due to inhibition of eicosanoid biosynthesis. In addition it may be effective in treating malaria, prevention of cervical cancer, and may interfere with the replication of the HIV virus. In HIV, it appears to act by interfering with P300/CREB-binding protein (CBP). It is also hepatoprotective. A 2008 study at Michigan State University showed that low concentrations of curcumin interfere with Herpes simplex virus-1 (HSV-1) replication. The same study showed that curcumin inhibited the recruitment of RNA polymerase II to viral DNA, thus inhibiting the transcription of the viral DNA. This effect was shown to be independent of effect on histone acetyltransferase activities of p300/CBP. A previous (1999) study performed at University of Cincinnati indicated that curcumin is significantly associated with protection from infection by HSV-2 in animal models of intravaginal infections.

Curcumin acts as a free radical scavenger and antioxidant, inhibiting lipid peroxidation and oxidative DNA damage. Curcuminoids induce glutathione S-transferase and are potent inhibitors of cytochrome P450.

A 2004 UCLA-Veterans Affairs study involving genetically altered mice suggests that curcumin might inhibit the accumulation of destructive beta-amyloid in the brains of Alzheimer's disease patients and also break up existing plaques associated with the disease.

There is also circumstantial evidence that curcumin improves mental functions; a survey of 1010 Asian people who ate yellow curry and were between the ages of 60 and 93 showed that those who ate the sauce "once every six months" or more had higher MMSE results than those who did not. From a scientific standpoint, though, this does not show whether the curry caused it, or people who had healthy habits also tended to eat the curry, or some completely different relationship.

Numerous studies have demonstrated that curcumin, amongst only a few other things such as high impact exercise, learning, bright light, and antidepressant usage, has a positive effect on neurogenesis in the hippocampus and concentrations of brain-derived neurotrophic factor (BDNF), reductions in both of which are associated with stress, depression, and anxiety.

Curcumin has also been demonstrated to be a selective monoamine oxidase inhibitor (MAOI) of type MAO-A.

In 2009 an Iranian group demonstrated the combination effect of curcumin with 24 antibiotics against Staphylococcus aureus.It is showed that in the presence of sub-inhibitory concentration of curcumin the antibacterial activities of cefixime, cefotaxime, vancomycin and tetracycline have been increased against test strain. Increase in inhibition zone surface area for these antibiotics were 52.6% (cefixime), 24.9% (cephotaxime), 26.5% (vancomycin), 24.4% (tetracycline). Also it is showed that curcumin has the antagonist effect on the antibacterial effect of Nalidixic acid against test strain.

Although many pre-clinical studies suggest that curcumin may be useful for the prevention and treatment of several diseases, the effectiveness of curcumin has not yet been demonstrated in randomized, placebo-controlled, double-blind clinical trials.

Its potential anticancer effects stem from its ability to induce apoptosis in cancer cells without cytotoxic effects on healthy cells. Curcumin can interfere with the activity of the transcription factor NF-κB, which has been linked to a number of inflammatory diseases such as cancer.

A 2009 study suggests that curcumin may inhibit mTOR complex I via a novel mechanism.

Another 2009 study on curcumin effects on cancer states that curcumin "modulates growth of tumor cells through regulation of multiple cell signaling pathways including cell proliferation pathway (cyclin D1, c-myc), cell survival pathway (Bcl-2, Bcl-xL, cFLIP, XIAP, c-IAP1), caspase activation pathway (caspase-8, 3, 9), tumor suppressor pathway , death receptor pathway (DR4, DR5), mitochondrial pathways, and protein kinase pathway (JNK, Akt, and AMPK)"

When 0.2% curcumin is added to diet given to rats or mice previously given a carcinogen, it significantly reduces colon carcinogenesis (Data from sixteen scientific articles reported in the Chemoprevention Database).

Little curcumin, when eaten, is absorbed: from 2 to 10 grams of curcumin eaten alone resulted in indetectable to very low serum levels. Curcumin is unstable in the gut, and the traces that pass through the GI tract rapidly degrade or are conjugated through glucuronidation.

Incorporating turmeric into the western diet poses challenges. A majority of Americans equate the mild-flavored turmeric with spicy Indian food. Most recipes incorporating turmeric, such as curries, are too spicy for many Americans because they contain hot spices such as cayenne pepper. There have been several commercial products developed to provide an alternate route to curcumin. For example, curcumin supplements with piperine are readily available. But curcumin in a non-solubilized pill form can limit bioavailability. Other products, such as Nutmeric, provide curcumin in an oil-solubilized form similar to Indian curry preparations. Co-supplementation with 20 mg of piperine (extracted from black pepper) significantly increased the absorption of curcumin by 2000% in a study funded by a prominent manufacturer of piperine. However, the increase in absorption only occurred during the first hour, after which the difference between the piperine curcumin and the regular curcumin was almost the same as far as absorption. Due to its effects on drug metabolism, piperine should be taken cautiously (if at all) by individuals taking other medications.

Some benefits of curcumin, such as the potential protection from colon cancer, may not require systemic absorption. Alternatively, dissolving curcumin in hot water or in warm oils prior to ingestion may possibly increase bioavailability; however, no published studies to date have documented this. Cooking with curcumin and oil may increase absorption, but peer-reviewed scientific literature has not documented this, while the literature has documented concerns regarding the heat stability of curcumin and its degradation in the gut.

In 2007, a polymeric nanoparticle-encapsulated formulation of curcumin ("nanocurcumin") has been synthesized which has the potential to bypass many of the shortcomings associated with free curcumin, such as poor solubility and poor systemic bioavailability. Nanocurcumin particles have a size of less than 100 nanometers on average, and demonstrate comparable to superior efficacy compared to free curcumin in human cancer cell line models. However, actual in vivo absorption has not been demonstrated with this nanoparticle.

In July 2008, researchers from the aforementioned team in UCLA's Department of Neurology announced results on a form of "lipidated curcumin" that was noted to achieve more than 5 micromolar in the brain in vivo, 50 times that found in clinical studies. Another method to increase the bioavailability of curcumin was filed in a patent in 2006. and involves a simple procedure creating a complex with soy phospholipids; the plasma concentration of curcumin using this method increased by 5-fold reaching 33.4 nanomolar in comparison to 6.5 nanomolar obtained with an equal molar quantity of unformulated curcumin administered as control.

Kawanishi et al. (2005) remarked that curcumin, like many antioxidants, can be a "double-edged sword" where in the test tube, anti-cancer and antioxidant effects may be seen in addition to pro-oxidant effects. Carcinogenic effects are inferred from interference with the p53 tumor suppressor pathway, an important factor in human colon cancer. Carcinogenic and LD50 tests in mice and rats, however, have failed to establish a relationship between tumorogenesis and administration of curcumin in turmeric oleoresin at >98% concentrations. Other in vitro and in vivo studies suggest that curcumin may cause carcinogenic effects under specific conditions.

In animal studies, hair loss (alopecia) and lowering of blood pressure have been reported. Clinical studies in humans with high doses (2–12 grams) of curcumin have shown few side effects, with some subjects reporting mild nausea or diarrhea. More recently, curcumin was found to alter iron metabolism by chelating iron and suppressing the protein hepcidin, potentially causing iron deficiency in susceptible patients. Further studies seem to be necessary to establish the benefit/risk profile of curcumin.

There is no or little evidence to suggest that curcumin is either safe or unsafe for pregnant women. However, there is still some concern that medicinal use of products containing curcumin could stimulate the uterus, which may lead to a miscarriage, although there is not much evidence to support this claim. According to experiments done on rats and guinea-pigs, there is no obvious effect (neither positive, nor negative) on the pregnancy rate, number of live or dead embryos.

Fo-Ti

It is the root of fo ti that is used for medicinal purposes and as a dietary supplement. In traditional Chinese medicine, fo ti is prepared by boiling it in an infusion made with black beans. The result is known as red fo ti, or processed fo ti. Red fo ti is thought to act as a tonic that improves energy and vitality, and is also thought to fortify the blood, liver and kidneys. The raw and unprocessed root is known as white fo ti.

Fo ti was first recorded in Chinese medicine in 713 AD during the Tang dynasty. He shou wu, translates to Chinese as "black-haired Mr. He". The name comes from an old Chinese legend. The story goes that an old villager called Mr. He was 58 and had been unable to father a child. He took fo ti on a regular basis after taking advice from a monk. The story goes that taking the root restored his youthful appearance (including his black hair) and his vitality. He was also able to father numerous children.

In Chinese medicine therefore, fo ti has been used to prolong life, cure premature graying and as a general cure for weakness. It has also been used to cure erectile dysfunction, vaginal discharge and constipation.

There is some scientific evidence that white fo ti can decrease serum cholesterol, assist with preventing hardening of the arteries, and can help boost immune function. There is also some evidence that suggests that fo-ti might improve memory and learning and reduce the degeneration of nigrostriatal dopaminergic neurons in the brain.

It has been shown in some studies on animals that fo-ti can reduce cholesterol in the blood. Fo ti contains lectins. In studies it has been shown that lectins may prevent the accumulation of cholesterol in the liver and may also prevent the retention of fat in the blood. Animal experiments have also shown that fo ti can assist in reducing the formation of fat deposits and plaque on arterial walls. Fo ti can also reduce the growth of bacteria, and has been shown to increase the ability of laboratory animals to adapt to cold conditions. It also promotes the production of red blood cells. Fo ti has also been shown to have an anti-tumor effect and acts as an antioxidant. The unprocessed fo ti roots can have a lubricating effect on the bowels, which in turn will have a laxative effect. A number of scientific studies carried out in China show that processed fo ti may be helpful in treating heart conditions, high cholesterol and chronic bronchitis.

Fo ti may be consumed as a whole root or sliced root. It may also be prepared as a powder, in capsule or tablets form and as a tincture. Most fo ti products on the market contain white fo ti, or the unprocessed root. The unprocessed root is usually a light brown color while red fo ti (cured or processed) is usually a dark reddish brown.

Is also indicated to boost the immune system and increase sexual vigour.

Chung Yun, a famous Chinese herbalist who reportedly lived to be 256 years old, used

Fo-Ti on a daily basis. This herb is thought to have been responsible for both his long life and his legendary sexual prowess, (he was said to have had 24 wives). In another Chinese legend Fo-ti was thought to be responsible for returning natural black colour to a previously gray-haired man- He Shou Wu means "black haired Mr. He." Thankfully, we have a little more to go on than folk medicine legends. Modern research indicates that this herb contains an alkaloid that has rejuvenating effects on the nerves, brain cells and endocrine glands. It stimulates a portion of the adrenal gland and helps to detoxify the body. Hair health, energy and sexual vigor are the products of this rejuvenation. Processed fo-ti contains protein-sugar complexes known as lectins. Processed fo-ti contains protein-sugar complexes known as lectins. Because they attach to specific arrangements of carbohydrates on cells in the body, lectins act like antibodies, but they do not cause allergy symptoms. The lectins in processed fo-ti may affect fat levels in the blood, helping to prevent or delay heart disease by blocking the formation of plaques in blood vessels. Plaques are accumulations of fat and other cells that restrict the size of blood vessels and limit the flexibility of their walls.

Latin Name: Polygonum multiflorum Common Names: Chinese Knotweed, Climbing Knotweed, Flowery Knotweed, He-Shou-Wu, Kashuu Properties: Astringent, demulcent, tonic. Uses: Atherosclerosis, Constipation, Fatigue, High cholesterol, Hair Health, Rejuvenation, Sexual Vigour, Detox the body, Lower cholesterol and blood pressure Indicated for: Blood deficiency, premature graying of the hair, nerve damage, wind rash, eczema, sores, carbuncles, goiter, scrofula and inflammation of lymph nodes and heat toxicity. Immune boosting.

Black Walnut Tincture

Walnut tincture is revered for its use in both human and animal medical care. A tincture is described as being between 40-60% of alcohol that has been infused with either oils or hulls. With a black walnut tincture, the black walnut is left intact and then soaked in alcohol. It is recommended that black walnuts be at least 50% green when selected for the infusion process. Sometimes, vitamin c or other ingredients might be added to the tincture.

However, the basis of all tinctures is alcohol. When the walnuts are soaking, it is recommended that they be covered entirely in alcohol. They are usually left between three days and three weeks to ensure that the walnut tincture is strong and potent. There are several ways to create a tincture. Due to the type of alcohol that is used in the preparation of tinctures, it may or may not be suitable for internal use. Always read the manufacturer's label to determine if the walnut tincture you are using is recommended for only external, or both internal and external use.

The scientific name for black walnut is Juglans Nigra. It is also referred to as the American Walnut. The black walnut tree grows from the southern most parts of Canada to the most southern tips of both Florida and Texas. It is native to the eastern parts of North America, but has been introduced into European regions. It is a hardy tree that grows to heights reaching between 100 and 130 feet.

Walnut tincture is an important aspect of herbal medicine, and has been used for thousands of years. There are many conditions that both the medical and alternative medical community treats on a regular basis. The idea of alternative medicine or using non-traditional methods to cure illness and disease is often a controversial topic. For those who have found success with herbs and alternative medicine, there is no doubt that the use of a walnut tincture is prevalent. From the early Romans to the middle ages, walnut has played a vital role in helping to treat a variety of conditions and illnesses. There are two main ingredients in walnuts that are attributed with the plants healing abilities. The first is juglone and the second is tannins. Juglone is rich in all parts of the black walnut, from the leaves and bark to the nut. This chemical is very strong and is toxic to other plants. In fact when the black walnut tree grows in the wild, it is often solitary or separate from many other species as to the high toxicity level of the Juglone in the tree. However, there are certain grasses that thrive by being in close proximity to the walnut tree. Because Juglone has a high toxicity level, it is also strong for the purpose of healing. Juglone is powerful for treating parasites, intestinal worms, fungus, and is even being used in a treatment for cancer. Thought the FDA doesn't regulate the use of herbs or monitor their effectiveness, they are often used with great success by alternative health practitioners.

The other chemical that makes black walnut a powerful herb in the fight against sickness and disease is tannins. Plants and trees to protect them from parasitic invasions and bacteria use tannins. Tannins are readily abundant in a wide variety of fruits, nuts, seeds, berries, and herbs. They hold great use for animal and human health as they help the body build resistance to bacteria and parasites. They are also found in tea and wine and have a direct impact on why these drinks are known for their health giving properties. Tannins are polyphenols, at one point; they were referred to as Vitamin P. Polyphenols are antioxidants, and you can rest assured that when you take a walnut tincture you are getting all of the same benefits of an antioxidant.

In addition to Juglone and tannins, black walnut is also high in chromium and iodine. Iodine is highly antiseptic and helps stimulate the function of the thyroid. The affects of iodine on energy levels have been proved and it can help increase mental awareness and lessen the effects of fatigue and depression. Iodine will also attack harmful bacteria and helps strengthen the immune system. It is the combination of these chemicals that make a walnut tincture such a vital tool in the fight against sickness.

If you are receiving medical treatment for a condition and are considering using black walnut tincture you should discuss this with your health care provider. Though walnut is a natural compound, there can be reactions with other vitamins, minerals, herbal supplements, or prescription medication. Always speak to your health care provider and make certain that you let him or her know of any herbal remedies, tinctures, or other preparations that you are taking.

Many people make the mistake of believing that just because something is natural it isn't powerful or potentially harmful. It is because herbal remedies are so powerful, that they can apply those properties against bacteria, fungi, and germs. You must let your health care provider know of everything that you take, including over the counter remedies, herbal preparations and formulas, and vitamins and mineral supplements.

Black walnut is known for its antiseptic, germicidal, and anti parasitic properties. It also works for many digestive orders. It can be applied topically, in the form of a walnut tincture or oil and is used for treating skin conditions that are the result of infection, fungus, or bacteria. It has been successful in treating athlete's foot, yeast or candida, ringworm, and thrush. Other skin conditions that have shown good response to black walnut tincture include psoriasis and eczema.

Internally, black walnut is used for removing parasites from the intestines and helps to regulate thyroid function. It removes worms from both humans and pets and has been used for treating parasitic conditions in dogs, cats, and horses. Additionally, many have found that regular treatment with black walnut can also assist in weight loss, as it is believed to balance glucose levels. Remember that it is important to read the label on any walnut tincture you purchase to ensure whether or not it can be taken internally.

Hawthorne Berry

Hawthorn herbs come from the Hawthorne Berry, which is a small red berry that looks like a miniature apple as it too grows on a tree. This thorny tree grows 30 feet tall and has beautiful pink or white flowers during the spring. There is a good reason why Hawthorne Berries are used as heart disease herbs. Not only can they help to regulate your blood pressure but they can also break down cholesterol and fat, both of which contribute to heart disease. They also help dilate coronary blood vessels so that your body is able to utilize oxygen, blood and nutrients more efficiently throughout your entire body. Hawthorne Berry is loaded with bioflavanoids, which are potent antioxidants. In fact, there are a lot of people who believe that they are actually a lot more potent than Vitamins A, C or E. It is these bioflavanoids that help your heart muscle be able to pump blood more efficiently. Whenever you have healthy arteries you will also have more endurance, good blood pressure and healthy blood vessels. This is the reason why this natural heart medicine is actually best used as a preventative medicine but it can also be used to treat heart disease too.

The vascular system is also important whenever it comes to supporting your heart. It has been shown that Hawthorne Berry will reduce calcification of your vascular system. As such, this heart extract will stop the arteries that lead to your heart from hardening or narrowing. You also won't develop any blot clots, which can lead to strokes and heart attacks.

Hawthorne Berry tea is often used for natural heart health even today. It can be made from the berries, the berry leaves or even the flowers of this herb. This tea is packaged and sold at most health food stores throughout the world. You can also get this alternative medicine for the heart in capsules or as a tincture.

Ever since the early 1900's, and even continuing today, there have been clinical trials and research done in regard to the medicinal value of Hawthorne Berry extract. Unfortunately, science has only partially evaluated the benefits of this herb on human health though. Nevertheless, it is still believed that the antioxidants, flavanoids and other compounds that are found in the Hawthorne Berry give this herb its beneficial effects. For this reason, it is sometimes added to heart herbal remedies in order to help reduce a person's blood pressure and correct any potentially unhealthy cholesterol levels.

Recently most of the studies about Hawthorne Berry extract are concerned with the medicinal value of this extract in regard to its affect upon a person's liver, digestive system and cardiovascular system. Many of these studies are also looking at Hawthorne Berry as an anti-inflammatory agent. The many studies that have been completed thus far have not looked at the use of Hawthorne Berry tea so much as they have looked at the usage of the concentrated extract itself.

While there are some health care professionals who have recognized the medicinal value of Hawthorne Berry extract for more than 100 years now, research on this extract is still considered to be only preliminary.

Hawthorne berries are thought to be one of the safest herbal heart supplements on the market today. As with any other medication, Hawthorne berries do have some side effects that occur on rare occasions. These include headaches, nausea and rapid heartbeat. It is also important to understand that there are a few possible drug interactions too. Therefore, if you are taking any prescription medications, you should contact your doctor before taking.

False Unicorn

False unicorn or liatris was used in colonial times for medicinal purposes, but now is almost an ornamental. Florists favor it when making cut flower arrangements for some of their customers because of its lovely lavender spikes of feathery flowers. Unlike most other spike flowers, this one is an exception to the rule and flowers from the top of the spike downward. The flower spikes may reach 2 feet or longer and can be either lavender or purple. False unicorn has great medicinal use.

False unicorn is used to treat venereal disease, especially gonorrhea. A small piece of the root is cleaned, finely chopped and simmered in 3 cups boiling water for 20 minutes.

After the liquid has sufficiently cooled, it is then strained and used both as a vaginal douche and wash to get rid of this infection.

Sore throats are quite common during cold and flu seasons. But sometimes they can get so bad that the breath develops an offensive smell. To eliminate this problem, just gargle with some tea made from false unicorn root every hour, according to the previous instructions.

False unicorn root is another herb inherited from the Native American tradition. False unicorn contains hormone-like saponins, which partly account for its long tradition as an excellent ovarian and uterine tonic. False unicorn was used specifically for uterine weakness and over-relaxation, characterized by a dragging sensation, a feeling of downward pressure in the pelvis, often associated with irritability and depression. False unicorn has also been used to encourage fertility in women and treat impotence in men. False unicorn has an adaptogenic or balancing effect on sex hormones, helping to relieve many disorders of the reproductive tract, menstrual irregularities and premenstrual syndrome, which are related to hormonal imbalance. False unicorn improves the secretory responses and cyclical functions of the ovary and has been used in infertility caused by dysfunction in follicular formation in the ovary.

The bitter principle has a tonic effect on the liver and digestive tract, which benefits appetite and digestion and helps to relieve nausea and vomiting in pregnancy. False unicorn root has also been used to prevent threatened miscarriage and to stop hemorrhage.

Tortoise Shell

The tortoise (gui) is one of the four spiritually endowed creatures. Described in the Book of Rites of the Confucian Classics, where it serves as an emblem of strength, longevity, and endurance, and symbolizes the Universe. Each of these creatures is associated with a direction and element, the tortoise, usually depicted in conjunction with a snake, represents the north, and is thereby associated with the water, darkness (the color black), and the earth, the element which was later put into the five element system in the center. The tortoise shell was long used in divination, by observing the patterns of cracks that developed when a hot instrument was touched to one of its many "divination points," and then interpreting the implication of the pattern. The prognostications and insights learned from the cracks were often written right onto the shells, and it is from buried fragments of tortoise shells (along with some mammal bones that were used similarly) that we know the most ancient forms of Chinese writing. Two lines depicting cracks represent the Chinese character but, which means to divine by looking at the cracks in the tortoise shell as the heat develops them. This character became incorporated into numerous others as a radical. Thus, the tortoise and its shell have been an important part of Chinese culture.

Further, the tortoise has been used as both food and medicine since ancient times, and is recorded as being used for these purposes since the Han Dynasty, 2000 years ago. Regarding their inclusion in the Chinese diet, E. N. Anderson comments that "Animals that are very tenacious of life, or very unusual-looking and -acting, are regarded as having special power; they are supplementing (bu). Notable supplementing foods are pangolins, raccoon dogs, soft-shelled turtles, tortoises, snakehead fish, and birds of prey....

Although the tortoise is not a major food in China today (turtles have long been preferred over tortoises for food), it remains one of the foods included in some diets. Anderson also points out that "During Han, and throughout Chinese history, the boundary between medicine and food was so vague as to be non-existent in practice. Many things were purely medicines, but medicines often became foods if people learned to like them; many foods became merely medicines when people stopped relishing them...."

ANIMAL MEDICINES AND THEIR CONSTITUENTS

Tortoise shells were described as medicines in the Shennong Bencao Jing , listed there as guijia (tortoise scale). They have become one of the standard items of the Materia Medica, with consistent use since the earliest recorded medical books. In fact, shells, along with similar animal materials, such as scales, antlers, and skins, are the most commonly used animal substances in the Chinese Materia Medica. Among these, oyster shell is probably the most widely used, followed by deer antler, tortoise shell, and pangolin scale, with lesser amounts of donkey skin gelatin and turtle shell being utilized, though still important to Chinese practice. These materials are rich in collagen and calcium compounds; collagens are the proteins that help determine the overall physical structure and the calcium compounds contribute to rigidity. Pangolin scale, as well as other animal materials such as cicada slough, snake slough, and horns (rhino, antelope, buffalo), are comprised mainly of another protein, keratin, which is similar to collagen; turtle and tortoise shells, as well as deer antlers contain some keratin (the hairs of antler velvet are mainly keratin).

Oyster shell, which is extremely hard, is mainly comprised of calcium carbonates and calcium phosphates with relatively little protein, while donkey hide is mainly comprised of collagen with a little calcium; the other materials mentioned above have intermediate content (see Appendix 1 for an analysis of the roles of these two compounds). As an example, deer antler in velvet (which is the most studied item) contains about 50% protein, with about half of it in the form of collagen that can be converted to gelatin. It also contains calcium carbonate, calcium phosphate, and calcium chloride, making up about 50% of the antler, and the amount of those components increases as the antler ages and becomes ossified (hardened), with a decline in the amount of collagen and other proteins. Tortoise shell and deer antler also contain chondroitin sulfate, a protein-polysaccharide complex that has recently been utilized to treat joint degeneration (it is a building block of the cartilage, comprised mainly of glucosamine). Small amounts of cholesterol and other animal substances are also present in the shells, scales, and skins. An alcohol extract of deer antler (alcohol doesn't solubilize collagen or calcium), called pantocrine, is reported to have hemopoietic and androgenic activity; its ingredients have not been reported. Presumably, tortoise shell also contains some substances that contribute similar kinds of activity. A 70% alcohol extraction medium solubilizes 2–3% of the substances in tortoise and turtle shells (31). Traditionally, antler is said to tonify and open the governing vessel (dumai) while tortoise shell tonifies and opens the conception vessel (renmai), the two vessels that run along the midline of the body, back (yang) and front (yin), respectively. Perhaps there are slightly differing constituents that can be found to explain the differing attributes. The Chinese interpretation may have originated with the observation of the natural materials more than from observation of physiological responses: the antler arises from the back and top of the deer's head (yang) and the plastron protects the tortoise's underbelly (yin).

Tortoise shell, as a medicinal agent, is most often utilized in rehmannia-based formulas that nourish the yin and blood and settle the yang (5). Relatively little is known of the pharmacology of the individual herbs of these formulas, though the overall effects include changes in hormones and hormone receptors. It is possible that tortoise shell provides a nutritional component to some formulas, with calcium and protein, though the flesh of the tortoise would be a better source of protein. Until recently, oyster shell calcium was the main source for calcium in Western nutritional supplements (now, more absorbable forms are often used instead); these supplements are reputed to have several medicinal applications, especially for calcium-deficient individuals.

The use of animal substances, such as tortoise shell, in the modern practice of natural healing is somewhat unusual for Westerners, many of whom view herbalism as a practice involving only plant materials (whereas Chinese "herbs" include minerals and animals). Indeed, for many Westerners, the use of herbs as a standard part of health care is often allied with practices, such as vegetarian diet, that differ from standard Chinese approaches and that would eliminate from consideration the ingestion of animal-derived medicinals. The use of tortoise shell is of particular concern to Westerners because some tortoises have been placed on the endangered species list, and are thereby prohibited from collection and trade. The tortoise shells used in Chinese medicine are obtained from aquatic but land-based tortoises, which are not included on the endangered species list, unlike sea tortoises or some desert species. However, due to the modernization of China (including plans to install a major dam across the Yangzi River), along with its large and still growing population, even these land tortoises may become endangered in the future. Increasing efforts are being made in China (and elsewhere) to raise the tortoises.

Echinacea

Echinacea is Used For Colds, Pregnancy, and Other Health Problems

The Benefits Echinacea

Perhaps the most popular and well-known herb on the natural market today is called Echinacea. This is an herb that has been used for a number of years and it is currently one of the most popularly used herbal treatments. It is primarily used to treat upper respiratory infections, influenza and other common infectious diseases.

Echinacea Basics

Echinacea's most common name is the purple coneflower. In reality, however, it is an herb that is made up of nine different varieties. Three of these varieties are used in herbal medicine. These include:

*Echinacea purpurea

*Echinacea engustifolia

*Echinacea pallida

Much of the purple coneflower plant is used to make Echinacea, including the leaves, stems, roots and flowers. They are used in a wide variety of different natural products made from these parts. How the Echinacea is made plays a role in what it is used for and how much is used. Certain of the preparations are used for the treatment of immune system disorders, bacterial infections and viral infections.

Healing powers of Echinacea

There is reason to believe that Echinacea improves the healing process of skin wounds. It may also control inflammation. Among natural herbalists, Echinacea has been tried in the treatment of skin sores, inflammation, abscesses, eczema and canker sores. One can actually put the herb directly on the affected area or take it by mouth to achieve basically the same effect.

One uncommon use for Echinacea is that of the treatment of CFS or chronic fatigue syndrome. Not everyone has shown improvement; many of those with CFS have improved in their symptoms after using Echinacea.

You can purchase Echinacea in many formulations, including dried tablets, tinctures, soft gels and liquids. You can also get Echinacea in a simple dried form. This can be steeped in hot water to make a nutritious tea. There are even cream preparations of the herb that is used topically on sunburns and skin rashes.

Make sure you read the back of the label whenever you are purchasing Echinacea. You'll find that certain formulations will involve more than one variety of the purple coneflower, while others will be of just one variety. Choose the type of Echinacea in the formulation that best suits your particular need.

Hoodia Gordoni

What is Hoodia Gordonii?

Latin Name: Hoodia gordonii

Other Names: hoodia, xhooba, !khoba, Ghaap, hoodia cactus, South African desert cactus

Hoodia (pronounced HOO-dee-ah) is a cactus-like plant that grows primarily in the semi-deserts of South Africa, Botswana, Namibia, and Angola.

In the last few years, hoodia has been heavily marketed for weight loss and has become immensely popular.

Although there has always been a demand for diet pills, after the ban on the herb ephedra, the market was particularly ripe for the next new diet pill.

Much of hoodia's popularity stems from claims that the San Bushmen of the Kalahari desert relied on hoodia for thousands of years to ward off hunger and thirst during long hunting trips. They were said to have cut off the stem and eat the bitter-tasting plant.

Hoodia gordonii grows in clumps of green upright stems. Although it is often called a cactus because it resembles one, hoodia is actually a succulent plant.

It takes about five years before hoodia gordonii's pale purple flowers appear and the plant can be harvested.

There are over 13 types of hoodia. The only active ingredient identified so far is a steroidal glycoside that has been called "p57". Currently, only hoodia gordonii is thought to contain p57.

What is the History of Hoodia Gordonii?

In 1937, a Dutch anthropologist studying the San Bushmen noted that they used hoodia gordonii to suppress appetite. In 1963, scientists at the Council for Scientific and Industrial Research (CSIR), South Africa's national laboratory, began studying hoodia. They claimed that lab animals lost weight after they were given hoodia gordonii.

The South African scientists, working with a British company named Phytopharm, isolated what they believed to be an active ingredient in hoodia gordonii, a steroidal glycoside, which they named p57. After obtaining a patent in 1995, they licensed p57 to Phytopharm. Phytopharm has spent more than $20 million on hoodia research.

Eventually pharmaceutical giant Pfizer learned about hoodia and expressed interest in developing a hoodia drug. In 1998, Phytopharm sub-licensed the rights to develop p57 to Pfizer for $21 million. Pfizer returned the rights to hoodia to Phytopharm, who is now working with Unilever.

Much of the hype about hoodia started after 60 Minutes correspondent Leslie Stahl and crew traveled to Africa to try hoodia. They hired a local Bushman to go with them into the desert and track down some hoodia. Stahl ate it, describing it as "cucumbery in texture, but not bad." She reported that she lost the desire to eat or drink the entire day.

She also said she didn't experience any immediate side effects, such as indigestion or heart palpitations.

How Does Hoodia Gordonii Work?

Despite its popularity, there are no published randomized controlled trials in humans to show hoodia is safe or effective in pill form.

One study published in the September 2004 issue of Brain Research found that injections of p57 into the appetite center of rat brains resulted in altered levels of ATP, an energy molecule that may affect hunger. The animals receiving the P57 injections also ate less than rats that received placebo injections. However, this was an animal study and injections in the brain are different from oral consumption, so it cannot be used to show that oral hoodia can suppress appetite in humans.

The manufacturer Phytopharm cites a clinical trial involving 18 human volunteers that found hoodia consumption reduced food intake by about 1000 calories per day compared to a placebo group.

Astralagus

Huang qi, pak kei, yellow leader and milk vetch. Perennial plant, native to northern China and Mongolia, that bears small yellow flowers.It has a thick root with a yellowish, fibrous, tough skin that has a slightly liquorice taste.The dried roots, and extracts thereof are used. A Chinese herb with properties that strengthen vitality, stamina, disease resistance, and improve the ability to cope with physical and emotional stress.

It contains numerous triterpene saponins (astragalosides I-X, isoastragalosides I-IV and soyasaponin I) as well as polysaccharides (astragalan, astraglucan AMem-P) and isoflavones (calycosin and formononetin)

- **Internal use**
    - o Improves adrenal gland and digestive function.
    - o Strengthens and boosts the immune system by improving the ability of the macrophages (type of white blood cells) to fight and devour bacteria, fungi and viruses and is also thought to promote the production of interferon in the body.
    - o People with regular colds and flu can benefit from this herb as it helps to build up natural resistance.
    - o Cancer patients also benefit from astragalus, as the addition of this herb makes some cancer medication more effective, thereby allowing less toxic dosages to be used in treatment.

- It is further indicated for use by cancer patients undergoing chemotherapy and radiation as a supportive measure to prevent liver damage, as this herb exhibits good liver protecting qualities.
- It increases metabolism and encourages sweating, while promoting healing and providing energy to combat fatigue.
- A Chinese study has also indicated that the herb improves sperm motility (spontaneous motion), as well as reducing high blood pressure and enhancing the immune system.
- It helps to improve circulation after a heart attack and helps to protect the tissue in these cases as well.
- It has been found in tests to relieve angina pain without the side effects of medicine normally used for this purpose.
- As the herb is useful to treat bladder infections caused by Proteusbacteria, it is also of value in fighting the formation of kidney stones.
- In patients with diabetes it is used to improve not only blood flow but also helps improve fasting blood sugar levels.
- In China, the root is peeled and dried, covered in honey and sold as a sweet on a stick.

The herb should not be taken in the presence of fever or during an illness. It should rather be used when recuperating from an illness and to maintain good health.

People taking blood thinning medication, or beta-blocker medication should be careful when using this herb, as it may cause bleeding when taken together with warfarin and make beta-blockers less effective.

Goldenseal

Other names: Yellow root, Orange root, Puccoon, Ground raspberry, Wild curcuma

Goldenseal (Hydrastis canadensis) is one of the most popular herbs on the market today. It was traditionally used by Native Americans to treat skin disorders, digestive problems, liver conditions, diarrhea, and eye irritations. Goldenseal became part of early colonial medical care as the European settlers learned of it from the Iroquois and other tribes. Goldenseal gained widespread popularity in the early 1800s due to its promotion by a charismatic herbalist named Samuel Thompson. Thompson believed goldenseal to be a magical cure for many conditions. Demand for this herb dramatically increased, until Thompson's system of medicine fell out of popularity.

Over the years, goldenseal has gone through periods of popularity. There is currently great demand for goldenseal, which coupled with limited supply of wild-crafted sources, has driven the price of goldenseal up.

Goldenseal is available in nutritional supplement form. It is also available as a cream or ointment to heal skin wounds.

Goldenseal herbal tincture can be used as a mouthwash or gargle for mouth sores and sore throats. A tea made of goldenseal can also be used for this purpose

Why Do People Use Goldenseal?

Goldenseal is a bitter that stimulates the secretion and flow of bile, and can also be used as an expectorant. It also has strong activity against a variety of bacteria, yeast, and fungi, such as E. Coli and Candida.

Goldenseal is used for infections of the mucus membranes, including the mouth, sinuses, throat, the intestines, stomach, urinary tract and vagina.

Goldenseal is used for the following conditions:

minor wound healing

bladder infections

fungal infections of the skin

colds & flu

sinus and chest congestion

Goldenseal became the center of a myth that it could mask a positive drug screen. This false idea was part of a novel written by pharmacist and author John Uri Lloyd.

Side Effects and Safety

Goldenseal should not be taken by pregnant women. One of goldenseal's chief constituents, berberine, has been reported to cause uterine contractions and to increase levels of bilirubin. People with high blood pressure should not use goldenseal. Those with heart conditions should only use goldenseal under the supervision of a health professional.

The safety of goldenseal in nursing women, children, and people with kidney and liver disease is unknown.

Side effects are rare, but include irritation of the mouth and throat, nausea, increased nervousness, and digestive problems. The liquid forms of goldenseal are yellow-orange and can stain.

Asian ginseng

The name "ginseng" is used to refer to both American (Panax quinquefolius) and Asian or Korean ginseng (Panax ginseng), which belong to the species Panax and have a somewhat similar chemical makeup. Siberian ginseng or Eleuthero (Eleutherococcus senticosus), on the other hand, is an entirely different plant with different effects. It is distantly related to ginseng, but it does not contain the same active ingredients. Both Asian and American ginseng contains ginsenosides; substances that are thought to give ginseng its medicinal properties.

Like American ginseng, Asian ginseng is a light tan, gnarled root that often looks like a human body with stringy shoots for arms and legs. Thousands of years ago, herbalist's thought that because of the way ginseng looks it could treat many different kinds of ailments, from fatigue and stress to asthma and cancer. In traditional Chinese medicine, ginseng was often combined with other herbs and used often to bring longevity, strength, and wisdom to its users.

Ginseng is sometimes called an "adaptogen," an herb that helps the body deal with various kinds of stress, although there is no scientific evidence of adaptogens. But ginseng has been studied for several conditions, and it remains of the most popular herbs in the United States. Many of the studies examining Asian or Korean ginseng have used combinations of herbs, so it's not always possible to say whether ginseng alone had any benefit. Research on Asian ginseng has included the following:

Immune system health

Asian ginseng is believed to enhance the immune system, possibly helping the body fight off infection and disease. Several clinical studies report that Asian ginseng can improve immune function. Studies have found that ginseng seems to increase the number of immune cells in the blood, and improve the immune system's response to a flu vaccine. In one study, 227 participants received either ginseng or placebo for 12 weeks, with a flu shot administered after 4 weeks. The number of colds and flu were two-thirds lower in the group that took ginseng.

Cardiovascular health

Asian ginseng seems to have antioxidant effects, meaning it helps rid the body of free radicals, substances that can damage DNA and are thought to contribute to heart disease, diabetes, and other conditions. Preliminary studies suggest Asian ginseng may improve the symptoms of heart disease in humans. It also may decrease "bad" LDL cholesterol levels and raise "good" HDL cholesterol.

Its effect on blood pressure is more complicated. Some studies have found it seems to lower blood pressure, while others find it causes blood pressure to rise. That had led some people to theorize that ginseng may increase blood pressure at usual doses but lower it when doses are higher. Until researchers know for sure, you should not take ginseng if you have high blood pressure unless your doctor tells you it's OK.

Type 2 diabetes

Although American ginseng has been studied more for diabetes, both types of Panax ginsengs may lower blood sugar levels in those with type 2 diabetes. However, in a few studies it appeared that Asian or Korean ginseng worsened blood sugar levels. Some people think that the ginsenosides found in American ginseng might lower blood sugar while the different ginsenosides in Asian ginseng could raise blood sugar levels. Until more is known, you should not take ginseng if you have diabetes without your doctor's strict supervision and monitoring.

Mental performance

People who take ginseng often say they feel more alert. Several studies report that Asian ginseng may slightly improve thinking or learning. Early research shows that Asian ginseng may improve performance on such things as mental arithmetic, concentration, memory, and other measures. More research in this area, although not easy to do, would be helpful. Some studies have also found a positive effect with the combination use of Asian ginseng and Ginkgo biloba.

The studies have varied in what kinds of mental function they measured, making it hard to know exactly what the effects of ginseng are. For example, one study found an increase in the ability to think abstractly among those who took ginseng, but no change in their reaction time or concentration levels.

Physical endurance

There have been a number of studies using Asian ginseng for athletic performance in humans and laboratory animals. Results have been mixed, with some studies showing increased strength and endurance, others showing improved agility or reaction time, and others showing no effect at all. Nevertheless, athletes often take Asian ginseng to boost both endurance and strength. Asian ginseng was also found to reduce fatigue in a study of 332 patients.

Stress and well-being

Asian ginseng is sometimes called an "adaptogen," something that helps the body deal with stress, whether physical or mental. While that can be difficult to study, there is some evidence that ginseng (both Asian and American types) can improve quality of life -- although quality of life can be hard to measure, too. A study of 501 men and women living in Mexico City found significant improvements in quality of life measures (energy, sleep, sex life, personal satisfaction, well-being) in those taking Asian ginseng. Another well-designed study found that people taking a nutritional supplement with ginseng reported better quality of life than those taking the same supplement without ginseng.

Fertility/erectile dysfunction

Asian ginseng is widely believed to be capable of enhancing sexual performance, but there aren't many studies to back this up. In animal studies, Asian ginseng has increased sperm production, sexual activity, and sexual performance. A study of 46 men has also shown an increase in sperm count as well as motility. Another study in 60 men found that Asian ginseng increased libido (sex drive) and decreased erection problems.

Alzheimer's disease

Individual reports and animal studies indicate that Asian ginseng may slow the progression of Alzheimer's, decrease senility, and improve memory and behavior. Studies of large groups of people are needed.

Cancer

Several studies suggest that Asian ginseng may reduce the risk of some types of cancers. In one observational study, researchers followed 4,634 people for 5 years and found that those who took ginseng had lower risk of lung, liver, pancreatic, ovarian, and stomach cancer. However, the study could not rule out other factors being responsible for the lower risk of cancer (including eating habits). And it found that taking ginseng as few as 3 times a year led to a dramatic reduction in cancer risk, which is hard to believe. A number of studies have found that Asian ginseng seems to inhibit the growth of tumors, although researchers aren't yet sure how it might work in humans. More research is needed.

Menopausal symptoms

There have been only a few studies examining ginseng for menopausal symptoms. Two well-designed studies evaluating red Korean (Asian) ginseng suggest it may relieve some of the symptoms of menopause, improving mood (particularly feelings of depression) and sense of well-being. The ginseng product was used in combination with a vitamin and mineral supplement. But another double-blind, placebo-controlled study of 384 women found no effect.

Yohimbe

Scientific/medical name(s): Pausinystalia yohimbe, (Corynanthe yohimbe) Yohimbe is an evergreen tree native to western Africa, specifically the countries of Nigeria, Cameroon, Gabon, and the Congo. It can reach a height of 90 feet. The dried bark is used in folk and herbal remedies. The drug yohimbine hydrochloride (called yohimbine), is derived from yohimbe bark, and has been approved by the U.S. Food and Drug Administration (FDA) for prescription use only. Yohimbe bark has been used as an aphrodisiac for many years. It has been declared an unsafe herb in Germany because of such complications as increased heart rate and blood pressure and even kidney failure. In the United States, supplements that are labeled as containing yohimbe bark often contain very little of it. On the other hand, yohimbine hydrochloride, the substance in yohimbe bark thought to help with erections, is regulated as a prescription drug and is standardized to contain a precise amount of the labeled ingredient. It is mainly used as a treatment for erectile dysfunction (impotence), although there are concerns about its side effects and interactions with other medicines, alcohol, and even some foods. Yohimbine hydrochloride is often called simply yohimbine, although it is made under several brand names. Yohimbe bark extract is promoted as an aphrodisiac and sexual enhancer for men and women. Proponents say that yohimbe extracts are powerful antioxidants that can prevent heart attacks. Some also tout it is as a stimulant, antidepressant, and aid to weight loss. Yohimbine hydrochloride, often simply called yohimbine, is thought to be the most vital active ingredient of yohimbe bark. The drug yohimbine is available by prescription for the treatment of erectile dysfunction and is supposed to improve blood flow to the penis. It has also been promoted to treat exhaustion, drug overdose (from clonidine), and a form of low blood pressure that occurs when standing, called postural hypotension. Yohimbine can also be used to enlarge the pupil of the eye to help doctors examine the inside of the eyes. Yohimbe bark and bark extracts are sold as capsules, tablets, liquids, and powders. Some people make the bark into a tea, while others place the powdered bark under the tongue or sniff it. Extracts and supplements labeled as yohimbine that are sold in health food stores and over the Internet contain varying amounts of yohimbe and other ingredients. FDA researchers analyzed a number of commercial yohimbe bark products available over the counter. They found that the supplements contained less of the amount of yohimbine that would be found in actual yohimbe bark and also contained substances that do not occur in yohimbe bark. The FDA strictly regulates the prescription form of yohimbine. It is approved only for the treatment of impotence and is available in tablets and capsules. The standard dosage is 5.4 milligrams taken 3 times a day for no longer than 10 weeks. In Africa, yohimbe has been used for generations as an aphrodisiac and a treatment for erectile dysfunction. It was also used to treat fevers, leprosy, high blood pressure, and heart problems. In addition, warriors used it as a stimulant before battle. The powder was sometimes smoked to induce hallucinations, and yohimbe poultices were placed on the skin as an antiseptic and treatment for pain. In the 1890s, yohimbe began to be used medicinally in Europe. Yohimbe has been used to treat erectile dysfunction for more than 100 years. After manufacturers purified the substance called yohimbine hydrochloride from the tree's bark, it has been sold by prescription only in the United States. Yohimbe was in use by 1938, before new drugs were required to be reviewed and approved by the FDA. When stricter regulatory practices were introduced, sales of existing drugs were allowed to continue. Its popularity has decreased as sildenafil (Viagra) and similar drugs were approved starting in the late 1990s. Even with this decline in popularity, there is concern that over-harvesting because of yohimbe's popularity as a drug and dietary supplement is killing the yohimbe trees of Africa. Most clinical trials have looked at yohimbine, rather than at yohimbe bark. Clinical trials have found contradictions regarding the effectiveness of yohimbine for treating erectile dysfunction. The American Urological Association guidelines on treatment of erectile dysfunction state that it could not draw conclusions about yohimbine's effectiveness and safety and that larger studies are needed to evaluate it. A randomized clinical trial found that yohimbine may be a useful treatment for erectile dysfunction caused by psychological problems. Another randomized clinical study found that yohimbine was no better than a placebo as a first treatment for erectile dysfunction that had some physical basis. Other studies with yohimbine have shown it helps some with mild erectile problems, even those that have a physical basis. A review study concluded that yohimbine has a modest effect on erectile dysfunction caused by psychological factors, but not on erectile dysfunction due to physical causes. It appears that more research needs to be done to clarify the role of yohimbine in the treatment of erectile dysfunction. No studies to date have compared yohimbine to newer treatments for this problem. It is important to note that these studies were done using the drug yohimbine. Extracted chemicals are not the same as yohimbe bark. Studies of yohimbine would be expected to produce different results from studies using the raw plant. The unpurified plant extract would have different amounts of active compounds, more compounds that may cause unexpected effects, and many other differences. Yohimbine is now being used with other substances for the treatment of erectile dysfunction and may be helpful for men who cannot take the newer drugs for impotence. A 2002 study looked at yohimbine combined with L-arginine glutamate (a substance thought to affect erections), given to 45 men as a one-time dose 1 to 2 hours before intended sexual intercourse. Results showed that it worked better than placebo, although men with mild to moderate erectile dysfunction had more improvement than those with more severe problems. Yohimbine has also been tested in small studies with people who have low blood pressure and in those who faint after standing up. It appeared to be somewhat helpful, but more studies need to be done before it can be recommended for this use. Early studies have also suggested that it can dilate the pupil of the eye to help doctors examine the inside of the eye, but more information is needed. Several other drugs are available and widely used for that purpose by eye specialists. Yohimbine and yohimbe bark can increase heart rate and raise blood pressure. People who have high blood pressure; heart, kidney or liver disease; and anxiety or nervous disorders should not take yohimbe or yohimbine. Those who drink alcohol or take antidepressants, antipsychotic drugs, methadone, certain nausea medicines, or opioid pain medicines (such as morphine) should not use yohimbe or yohimbine. Other potential interactions between yohimbe and other drugs and herbs should be considered. Some of these combinations may be dangerous. Always tell your doctor and pharmacist about any herbs you are taking. Side effects of yohimbe bark or yohimbine include difficulty breathing, chest pain, palpitations, anxiety, queasiness, sleeplessness, and vomiting. Normal doses of yohimbine can cause a rise in blood pressure. Large doses of yohimbine (40 milligrams per day or more) can cause a drop in blood pressure and have been blamed for heart attacks and even deaths. Yohimbine can make heart disease or blood pressure problems worse. Less common side effects that do not usually require medical attention include dizziness, headache, flushing, nausea, nervousness, sweating, and tremors. People with emotional or psychiatric problems may have worsening of post-traumatic stress disorder, sleeplessness, and anxiety. New onset of panic attacks or manic episodes have been reported. Yohimbine has been linked to psychotic episodes. Yohimbine can also act as a monoamine oxidase inhibitor (MAOI), a type of powerful antidepressant. Foods that contain tyramine, such as beer, red wine, liver, aged or smoked meats, and aged cheese can raise blood pressure to dangerous levels if you eat them while taking yohimbine. Children, elderly people, or women who are pregnant or breast-feeding should not use yohimbine or yohimbe bark. Yohimbe bark is on the Commission E (Germany's regulatory agency for herbs) list of unapproved herbs. This means that it is not recommended for use because it has not been proven to be safe or effective. Relying on this type of treatment alone and avoiding or delaying conventional medical care for cancer may have serious health consequences.

Damiana

The ancient Mayan civilization utilized the damiana herb as a traditional aphrodisiac, and the people of Central America where the Mayan civilization was based utilize it to this day. As herbal tonic as well as an aphrodisiac, the damiana herb remains in continued use and is considered very valuable for its stimulatory action, as well as its tonic like effect on the body. This is the reason, that the herb action is such a valuable remedy for people affected by a mild depression to this day - herbalist will normally suggest the remedies made from this herb. The damiana herb is a very strong and aromatic herb, it has a slight bitter taste, and the leaves of the herb are used in countries such as Mexico to substitute for tealeaves and furthermore, the herb is also used as a flavoring agent for a variety of liqueurs.

Different preparations can be made from the leaves of the damiana herb, it can be taken in the form of an herbal tea or they can even be smoked like tobacco, the use of any of these derivatives will induce a relaxed state of mind in the individual using them. The herb will also induce a subtle kind of high tinged with sexual overtones, and the effect is a little reminiscent of the effects induced by smoking marijuana. Women are supposed to be much more highly effected by the medication especially, when they use it over a long period of time. Mexico produces some well-known damiana liqueurs, which are subtly advertised as aphrodisiacs, these liquids contain only very minute quantities of the herb, though they are reputed to be very effective. Moreover, the amount of herb infused into the liquor is sufficient, and give these beverages a distinctive herbal flavor.

Saw Palmetto

Other Common Names:
Sabal, Sabal Fructus, Fructus Serenoae, Sägepalmenfrüchte, Sägepalme.

Habitat:
Saw palmetto is found in sandy coastal lands or as undergrowth in pine forests in the

Southeastern United States.

Description:

Saw palmetto is a fan palm plant. The flowers produced by this plant are yellowish-white and the fruit is a reddish-black fleshy fruit with a pit.

Plant Parts Used:

The fruit. The Native Americans ate the fruit for nourishment but also used it for treatment of many urinary and genital disorders. The European settlers saw this use and developed additional uses for it. An extract from the fruit is used in herbal medicine today. Essential fatty acids and phytosterols are found in this extract. The fatty acids contained in saw palmetto are lauric acid, palmitic acid, oleic acid, and myristic acid. The polysaccharides; galactose, arabinose, and uronic acid, are also found in the fruit. Historically, saw palmetto has been used as a tea to treat benign enlargement of the prostate. It was commonly used to treat frequent urinary tract infections and it was also believed it could increase sex drive in men and sperm production. Frequent urination and excessive night urination, due to inflammation of the bladder or prostate, was a common condition treated by saw palmetto in the past.

Today many studies have been, and still are being, conducted on saw palmetto to test some of the common claims. It is commonly used today to tone the male reproductive system and boost the production in reproductive hormones in men. Females with fertility issues and reproductive organ problems have also used it as well. It is still being used to treat many urinary tract disorders. In some cases it has been shown to aid thyroid function and as a herbal remedy for asthma, bronchitis and other bronchial and throat problems, especially those related to excess mucous secretions. One of the other issues that its use has been focused on is benign prostatic hyperplasia (BPH.) Testosterone collects in the prostate and the converts to dihydrotestosterone (DHT.) This causes the cells to multiply quickly causing an enlargement of the prostate. Saw palmetto is thought to inhibit the conversion of testosterone to DHT and also the binding of DHT to receptor sites.

o Saw palmetto has also been touted as anabolic agent, contributing to muscle growth. This is also a by-product of the action on testosterone, stopping its conversion to DHT. This leads to more free-floating testosterone, which is an anabolic agent and leads to more muscle mass.

There are few, positive clinical trials published on the benefits of saw palmetto extracts both topically and internally as an herbal remedy for hair loss (baldness) in men.

Quinoa

Quinoa was of great nutritional importance in pre-Columbian Andean civilizations, being secondary only to the potato, and was followed in importance by maize. In contemporary times, this crop has become highly appreciated for its nutritional value, as its protein content is very high (12%–18%). Unlike wheat or rice (which are low in lysine), and like oats, quinoa contains a balanced set of essential amino acids for humans, making it an unusually complete protein source among plant foods. It is a good source of dietary fiber and phosphorus and is high in magnesium and iron. Quinoa is gluten-free and considered easy to digest. Because of all these characteristics, quinoa is being considered a possible crop in NASA's Controlled Ecological Life Support System for long-duration manned spaceflights.

Grape Seed Oil

Grapes (Vitis vinifera) have been heralded for their medicinal and nutritional value for thousands of years. Egyptians ate grapes at least 6,000 years ago, and several ancient Greek philosophers praised the healing power of grapes -- usually in the form of wine. European folk healers made an ointment from the sap of grapevines to treat skin and eye diseases. Grape leaves were used to stop bleeding, inflammation, and pain, such as the kind brought on by hemorrhoids. Unripe grapes were used to treat sore throats and dried grapes (raisins) were used for constipation and thirst. Round, ripe, sweet grapes were used to treat a range of health problems including cancer, cholera, smallpox, nausea, eye infections, and skin, kidney, and liver diseases.

But grapes -- or the chemicals within them, especially oligomeric proanthocyanidin complexes (OPCs) -- have been touted as powerful antioxidants. Some people believe they could help treat a number of conditions, from heart disease to cancer to aging skin, although scientific evidence is mostly lacking for those conditions. However, there is good evidence that grape seed extract can help treat chronic venous insufficiency and edema.

A study of healthy volunteers found that taking grape seed extract did substantially increase levels of antioxidants in their blood. Antioxidants are substances that destroy free radicals -- harmful compounds in the body that damage DNA (genetic material) and even cause cell death. Free radicals are believed to contribute to aging as well as the development of a number of health problems, including heart disease and cancer.

Plant Description:

Grapes are native to Asia near the Caspian Sea, but they were brought to North America and Europe around the 1600s. This plant's climbing vine has large, jagged leaves, and its stem bark tends to peel. The grapes may be green, red, or purple.

What's It Made Of?:

Vitamin E, flavonoids, linoleic acid, and OPCs are highly concentrated in grape seeds. These compounds can also be found in lower concentrations in the skin of the grape. OPCs are also found in grape juice and wine, but in lower concentrations. Resveratrol is another of grape's compounds which is related to OPCs and found mainly in the skins. Resveratrol has become very popular as an antioxidant and is being studied in connection with a variety of diseases.

Medicinal Uses and Indications:

Today, standardized extracts of grape seed may be used to treat a range of health problems related to free radical damage, including heart disease, diabetes, and cancer. Some studies -- mostly in animals -- support these uses.

Flavonoids found in red wine may help to protect the heart by lowering "bad" LDL cholesterol. The so-called "French paradox" is the belief that drinking wine protects people living in France from developing heart disease at the high rates seen in people living in the United States. So far, however, there is no clear evidence that taking grape seed extract helps reduce heart disease. Some researchers speculate that it may the alcohol in the wine, and not the flavonoids, that could be responsible for any healthful effects. Others think it could be the combination of alcohol and flavonoids.

Drinking alcohol to protect against heart disease is not advocated by the American Heart Association and other organizations because of the potential for addiction and other serious problems, such as car accidents and the increased risk of hypertension, liver disease, breast cancer, and weight gain. If you do drink red wine, you should have no more than 2 glasses (20 g ethanol) per day if you are a man, and no more than one if you are a woman.

Chronic venous insufficiency

In chronic venous insufficiency, blood pools in the legs, causing pain, swelling, fatigue, and visible veins. A number of high-quality studies have shown that OPCs from grape seed can reduce symptoms.

Edema

Edema -- swelling caused by surgery or an injury -- seems to go away faster when people take grape seed extract. Edema is common after breast cancer surgery, and one double-blind, placebo-controlled study found that breast cancer patients who took 600 mg of grape seed extract daily after surgery for six months had less edema and pain than those who took placebo. Another study found that people who took grape seed extract after experiencing a sports injury had less swelling than those who took placebo.

High cholesterol

There isn't enough evidence to say whether taking grape seed extract can lower cholesterol, although two preliminary studies showed promising results. A study of 40 people with high cholesterol looked at whether taking grape seed extract, chromium, a combination of both, or placebo for 2 months would lower cholesterol. The combination of grape seed extract and chromium was more effective than either grape seed alone or placebo in lowering total and LDL ("bad") cholesterol.

Another study looked at the effects of a proprietary grape seed extract on lipid peroxidation (the breakdown of fats in the blood) in a group of heavy smokers. Twenty-four healthy male smokers, (aged 50 years or greater) took either placebo or 2 capsules

(75 mg of a grape procyanidin extracts and soy-phosphatidalcholine), twice daily for 4 weeks. "Bad" LDL cholesterol levels were lower in those taking the grape seed supplement than those taking placebo.

High blood pressure

Theoretically, grape seed extract might help treat hypertension or high blood pressure. Antioxidants, like the ones found in grape seed, help protect blood vessels from damage. Damaged blood vessels can lead to higher blood pressure. In several animal studies, a grape seed extract substantially reduced blood pressure. But human studies are needed to see whether grape seed extract helps people with high blood pressure.

Cancer

Studies have found that grape seed extracts may prevent the growth of breast, stomach, colon, prostate, and lung cancer cells in test tubes. However, there is no clear evidence yet whether it works in humans. Antioxidants, such as those found in grape seed extract, are thought to reduce the risk of developing cancer. Grape seed extract may also help prevent damage to human liver cells caused by chemotherapy medications. Talk to your doctor or pharmacist before combining antioxidants with any chemotherapy drugs to make sure they interact safely together.

Other conditions

Grape seed extract is sometimes suggested for the following, although evidence is slight:

☐ Diabetes (improving blood sugar control)

 Improving night vision☐

☐ Protecting collagen and elastin in skin (anti-aging)

 Treating☐ hemorrhoids

Available Forms:

Grape seed is available as a dietary supplement in capsules, tablets, and liquid extracts. Look for products that are standardized to 40 - 80% proanthocyanidins or an OPC content of not less than 95%.

How to Take It:

Pediatric

Grape seed extracts are not recommended for children. Whole grapes, however, make a healthy and safe snack for children.

Adult

 To protect against free radical damage (oxidation), take☐ 25 - 150 mg of a standardized extract (40 - 80% proanthocyanidins or 95% OPC value), 1 - 3 times daily.

 Chronic venous insufficiency: 150 - 300 mg☐ daily

 Edema: 200 - 400 mg daily for 10 - 30 days☐

Precautions:

The use of herbs is a time-honored approach to strengthening the body and treating disease. Herbs, however, contain components that can trigger side effects and interact with other herbs, supplements, or medications. For these reasons, herbs should be taken with care, under the supervision of a health care provider qualified in the field of botanical medicine.

At the recommended dosage, grape seed is considered safe for up to 12 weeks. However, pregnant or breastfeeding women should not take grape seed supplements.

Possible Interactions:

There are no known scientific reports of interactions between grape seed and conventional medications. However, the OPCs in grape seed extract may interact with the following:

Anticoagulants (blood thinners) -- Grape seed extract may act as a blood-thinner, and could increase the risk of bleeding if taken with other blood-thinners such as warfarin (Coumadin). If you are taking blood thinning medications or have bleeding disorders, ask your doctor before taking grape seed extract.

Cooking

Grape seed oil has a high smoke point of approximately 216 °C (421 °F), so it can be safely used to cook at high temperatures, such as stir-frying, sautéing and deep-frying. Due to its clean, light taste, it is often used as an ingredient in salad dressings and mayonnaise and as a base for oil infusions of garlic, rosemary, or other herbs or spices. The metabolic energy density of grape seed oil is typical of vegetable oils: approximately 3,700 kJ (880 kcal) per 100 g, or 500 kJ (120 kcal) per 15 ml tablespoon. However, because less oil is needed for cooking, it can be used within a low-fat diet especially when combined with good frying techniques (such as using enough oil, not overcrowding the pan, and having the oil at the correct temperature), which reduces the amount of absorbed oil.

www.ingramcontent.com/pod-product-compliance
Lightning Source LLC
Chambersburg PA
CBHW081540280526
45788CB00010B/3304